CORNELIUS MULLER

Candida Clarity

A clear guide to a understanding Candida

Contents

I

Part One

1

Introduction

I f you are reading this you or somebody close to you is probably researching, diagnosed or battling with Candida. The ominous gut yeast bacteria that wrecks havoc and is notoriously difficult to kill off and cure. The word is almost shrouded in fear as diets to battle it range from Vegan, Gluten-Free, Keto to even Carnivore diet. For some a couple of weeks, others talk about months and so do the recovery stories. Well this book is here to cut the crap and demystify candida, give you as the reader an understanding of what exactly candida is, what its purpose is and how to kill overgrowth and ultimately how to fortify and balance the gut.

Candida is a type of yeast (fungus) that is part of the human microbial community. Candida albicans as it's formally known occurs in several areas of the body including the mouth, gastrointestinal tract, skin and genital areas. Candida overgrowth also known as candidiasis or yeast overgrowth is when the microbial balance in the body is compromised and allows Candida yeast to flourish beyond its normal level, which ultimately leads to several different health issues.

Candida overgrowth can occur in several different areas in the body namely gastrointestinal tract, skin and nail, genital areas, mouth &

tongue causing issue such as gas, bloating, brain fog, genital yeast infections, skin and infections and redness or rash and more seriously Candida overgrowth can spread beyond localized areas and enter the bloodstream, potentially leading to more serious systemic infections. The wide range of issues caused affect your overall well being too.

With such a wide ranging list of symptoms Candida is easily misdiagnosed or written off as just a simple infection etc and victims often live with it for months or years before it is accurately diagnosed and targeted. I say this because that is similar to what my own experience has been. Having recurring fungal infections on my skin, brain fog and bloating for years I always have written it off as isolated cases. That is until I had a wide spectrum health checkup and the Doctor pointed out I have a severe Candida overgrowth and that addressing Candida overgrowth often involves a multi-faceted approach, including dietary changes, lifestyle modifications, probiotics, antifungal treatments, and addressing any underlying health conditions. Bottom line treating Candida often involves a complete lifestyle and diet overhaul until you've killed it off or flushed it out so to say.

Now that we have a basic understanding of Candida, what it is and how we get an overgrowth it's time to dive into the book starting off with a more in-depth look into understanding Candida, an Overgrowth and the Candida-Diet connection.

2

The Candida Microorganism: An In-depth Overview

Candida Species and Varieties

Candida is a genus of yeast and even though it is *Candida albicans* that is most commonly associated with human health it is worth noting and knowing that the Candida yeast family comprises of various species, each with distinct characteristics and specific roles to play in the body and also different issues that may arise.

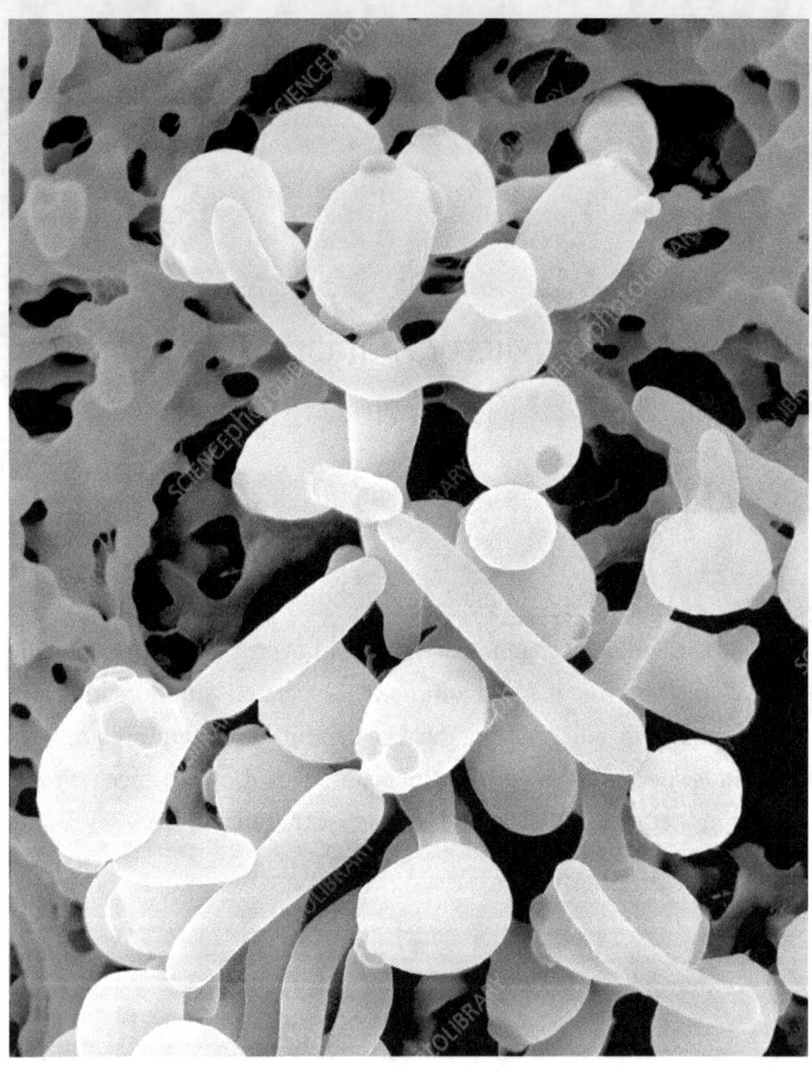

While there are over 20 different species of Candida identified and studied some of the more common and notable varieties are:

1. **Candida albicans:** The most prevalent species in the human body, found in the mouth, gastrointestinal tract, and genital area. It is both a commensal (beneficial in moderation) and an opportunistic pathogen (can cause infections under certain conditions).
2. **Candida glabrata:** Increasingly recognized as an opportunistic pathogen, often causing infections in individuals with compromised immune systems or those on long-term antibiotic therapy.
3. **Candida tropicalis:** Commonly associated with bloodstream infections and urinary tract infections.
4. **Candida parapsilosis:** Known for causing bloodstream and catheter-related infections, particularly in hospital settings.
5. **Candida krusei:** Exhibits intrinsic resistance to some antifungal drugs and is occasionally associated with infections in immuno-compromised individuals.
6. **Candida auris:** An emerging and often drug-resistant species responsible for healthcare-associated infections, with a particular concern due to its ability to spread rapidly in healthcare settings.

Candida's Role in the Body

Candida, when present in appropriate amounts, plays several important roles in the body's overall health and functioning:

1. **Microbial Balance:** Candida contributes to the balance of the body's microbial ecosystem, particularly in the gut, where it coexists with other beneficial bacteria. This balance is crucial for proper digestion, nutrient absorption, and immune function.
2. **Nutrient Recycling:** Candida helps break down and recycle nutrients in the digestive system, aiding in the digestion of complex carbohydrates and other substances.

3. **Protection Against Harmful Microbes:** Candida competes with potentially harmful microorganisms for space and resources in the gut, preventing their overgrowth and colonization.
4. **Immune Stimulation:** In controlled amounts, Candida interacts with the immune system, helping to maintain a balanced immune response and overall immune health.
5. **Biofilm Formation:** Candida can form biofilms, which are communities of microorganisms encased in a protective matrix. Biofilms have potential benefits in certain contexts, such as protecting against harmful bacteria, but they can also contribute to infections under certain conditions.

Understanding Candida's role in both health and disease is essential for effectively addressing Candida-related concerns and maintaining overall well-being.

3

The Candida Overgrowth Phenomenon

andida Overgrowth, also known as Candidiasis, is an extreme proliferation of the Candida yeast, primarily Candida albicans and is a complex and multifaceted condition.

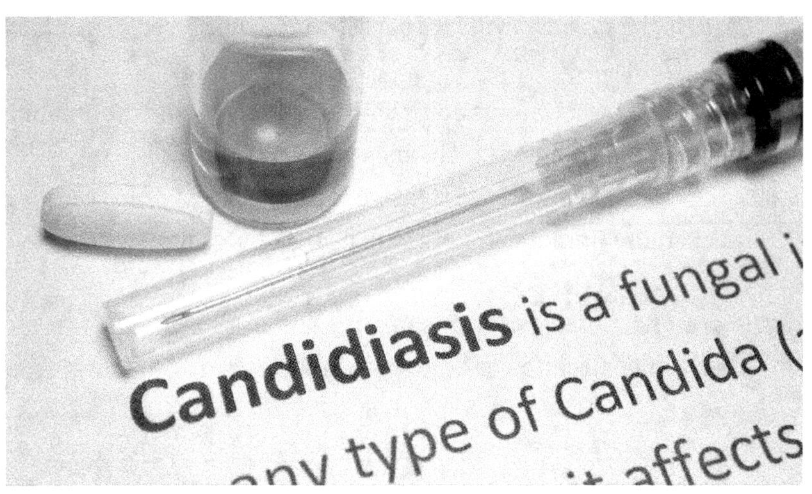

Often caused by a combination of factors upsetting the delicate balance of the microbial ecosystem Overgrowth can lead to a range of health issues both localized and systemic, affecting various body parts.

Factors leading to Candida Overgrowth:

Several factors can contribute to the development of Candida Overgrowth:

1. **Antibiotic use**: Broad spectrum Antibiotics can disrupt the balance of gut bacteria which allows Candida to multiply and thrive.
2. **Diet:** Diets high in refined sugar, carbohydrate and processed foods provide an abundant food source for the yeast.
3. **Alcohol Consumption:** Excessive alcohol consumption damage the gut lining and immune function allowing for a Overgrowth.
4. **Weakened Digestive Function:** Impaired digestion and gut motility leads to the stagnation of food particles providing breeding grounds for Candida.
5. **Chronic Stress:** Chronic or prolonged stress weakens the immune systems and the gut microbiome.
6. **Use of Corticosteroids:** Extensive use of Corticosteroids can also weaken the immune system which contributes to Candida overgrowth.
7. **Hormonal Changes:** Hormonal fluctuations such as during pregnancy, menstruation or hormonal therapies can also lead to overgrowth.

Signs and Symptoms Of Candida Overgrowth:

A wide variety of symptoms can manifest due to Candida Overgrowth and ranges from person to person. Some common Symptoms include:

1. **Digestive Issues:** Bloating, gas, diarrhea, constipation, and abdominal discomfort.
2. **Oral Thrush:** White patches on the tongue, inner cheeks, and throat, often accompanied by discomfort or pain.
3. **Vaginal Yeast Infections:** Itching, burning, and abnormal discharge in women.
4. **Skin Problems:** Skin rashes, itching, redness, and fungal infections like athlete's foot or nail fungus.
5. **Fatigue and Brain Fog:** Persistent fatigue, lack of energy, and difficulty concentrating.
6. **Mood Swings:** Mood disturbances, irritability, and anxiety.
7. **Recurrent Infections:** Frequent urinary tract infections or respiratory infections.
8. **Food Cravings:** Strong cravings for sugary and carbohydrate-rich foods.
9. **Joint Pain:** Unexplained joint pain and stiffness.

It's important to note that these symptoms can be from various causes and proper diagnosing is essential, which we will get into further in the book.

4

Exploring the Candida-Diet Connection

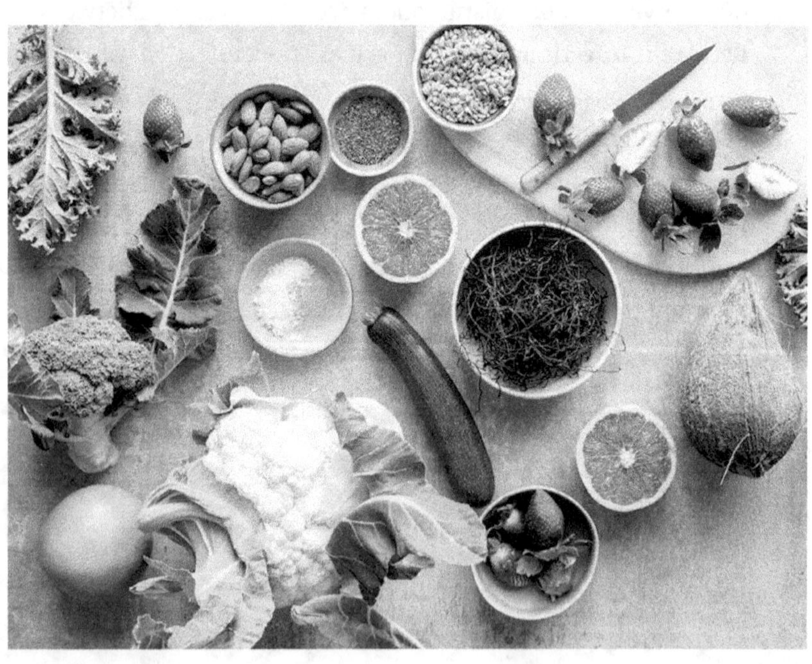

The Candida diet is the cornerstone to a Candida protocol, designed to starve and prevent the Candida from overgrowing by restricting its food sources and creating an unfavorable environment for it. While the diet plays a critically important role it is recommended to use it in conjunction with other strategies.

Understanding the Candida Diet:

The Candida diet focuses primarily on a couple of key principles namely:

1. **Limiting or removing Sugars:** Sugars and refined carbohydrates are the primary food sources for Candida. A typical Candida diet restricts the consumption of sugary foods including desserts, sugary snacks, sweetened drinks/beverages and in extreme cases fruit and high sugar vegetables.

2. **Reducing Processed foods:** Processed and heavily refined foods often contain hidden sugars and other additives that can contribute to candida overgrowth. These foods are minimized or preferably completely eliminated from the diet.

3. **Emphasizing Whole foods:** Whole foods like vegetables, lean proteins, healthy fats and for some whole grains are emphasized on the candida diet as they are nutrient-dense and unrefined.

4. **Including Anti-fungal foods:** Certain foods with antifungal properties such as: Coconut oil, garlic, ginger, oregano and certain mushrooms are included to help combat candida.

5. **Probiotic-Rich Foods:** Fermented foods like yogurt, kefir, sauerkraut, and kimchi are rich in pre & probiotic foods and support the gut microbiome so may be included, however they are often excluded initially in the reset of die off period.

6. **Avoiding Allergens:** Foods that commonly trigger sensitivities or allergic reactions like gluten, soy and dairy, may be eliminated to

help reduce inflammation and support the gut.

How Diet Influences Candida Overgrowth

What you put into your body could either feed candida or attack it and what you remove from your diet could either starve it or help your body in another way. Diet plays a critical role in Candida Overgrowth for several reasons.

Sugar feeds the candida, refined carbohydrates easily breaks down into sugars too and a diet high in these foods will contribute to Candida growth and overpopulation. Processed foods and allergens lead to inflammation in the gut and weakens your immune system's ability to control Candida. If your diet is lacking in essential nutrients it further weakens your immune system. So a diet that is full of nutrient dense whole foods, rich in fiber, probiotics and promotes a diverse and balanced microbiome all helps fight Candida.

It's very important to approach your diet with careful consideration and preferable under guidance of a nutrition expert or healthcare professional. While changing your diet is essential to managing Candida overgrowth individual needs vary and it may not be suitable for everyone. A holistic approach that includes dietary changes, lifestyle modifications and if necessary other medical interventions is the most effective strategy for addressing Candida.

II

Diagnosis and Assessment

5

Identifying Candida Overgrowth

Now that we know a bit more about Candida itself let's see how to identify Candida overgrowth. Candida overgrowth will elicit different responses from person to person and with symptoms differing even further depending on which body part is affected. If you suspect that you have a Candida overgrowth a thorough personal inspection is necessary and then to seek out professional healthcare advice. There are several different test protocols healthcare specialists can use to identify Candida and to pinpoint where and what type of candida even though as mentioned before most tests will be looking for Candida Albicans specifically. So let's dive into the topic of diagnosing Candida.

Self-Assessment and Symptoms Tracking

Self-assessment and symptom tracking play crucial roles in understanding and managing Candida-related issues. By consistently evaluating how you feel and noting any physical or emotional changes, you create a valuable record of your health journey. Tracking symptoms such as digestive disturbances, skin concerns, fatigue, and mood fluctuations enables you to identify patterns and potential triggers. This self-awareness empowers you to make informed decisions about dietary adjustments, lifestyle modifications, and seeking professional guidance when needed. Monitoring your body's responses and progress fosters a proactive approach to your well-being and aids in tailoring effective strategies for Candida management. If any of the symptoms are present and persist then seeking professional help is essential.

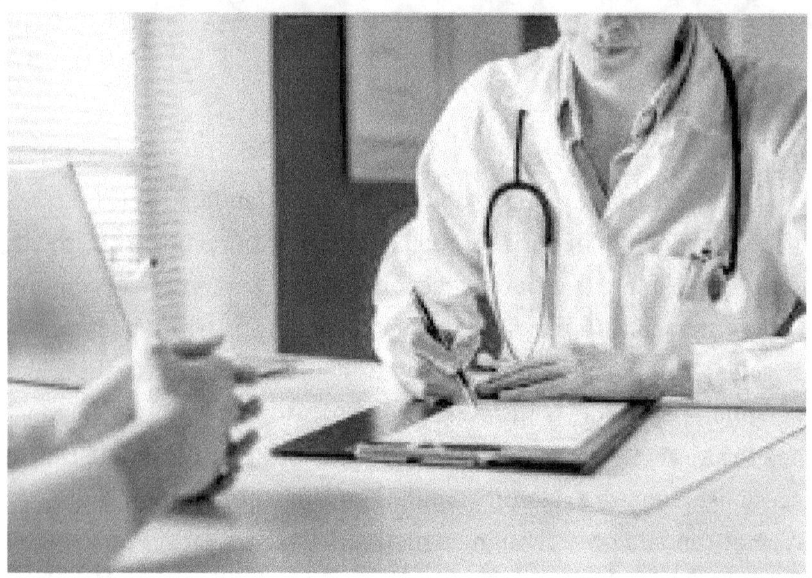

Medical Tests and Diagnostic Tools

Many Candidiasis symptoms overlap other health conditions issues and so it might be difficult to establish whether Candida is the cause or not. Your first indicators of Candidiasis like redness, itchy rashes, bloating, head fog can be many other issues and so it is important to get testing done to pinpoint and confirm the cause. Your healthcare provider will most likely take an approach of some of these medical tests below to safely determine the cause and potentially the extent of the overgrowth, variety and area of the body affected.

Common medical tests for candida:

1. **Skin Scrape**: This test serves as a screening method for detecting fungal skin or nail infections, without specifying the exact fungus. Common fungal infections include ringworm, athlete's foot, jock itch, and Candida. Cutaneous Candida, or Candidiasis of the skin, typically leads to a red, scaly, and itchy rash, mainly in skin folds like armpits, groin, finger spaces, nail edges, under breasts, and mouth corners.During a skin scrape test, a specialized tool is employed by a healthcare provider to extract a small skin or nail sample, which is then analyzed in a laboratory.

2. **Swab/Culture**: This test is specifically used for Candidiasis of the mouth or of the vaginal tract, also known as Thrush or Vaignal yeast infection respectively. A medical swab is used to collect tissue or fluid from the affected area and sent of to a lab to identify the type of fungal infection. Thrush will typically cause a whiteness of the tongue & cheeks, sores, redness and swelling. Vaginal yeast infections are identified by redness, swelling, pain during intercourse or urination and might give off a almost curd like substance.

3. **Urine/Uric Acid:** The organic acids test uses urine to measure compounds and waste products, providing a "metabolic snapshot" of overall health. Test kits from healthcare providers allow convenient home collection, then samples are sent to labs. Candida overgrowth in the gut produces metabolic waste that appears in urine as organic acids. For instance, D-arabinitol indicates yeast

overgrowth. Arabinose is another acid used for reference, but dietary restrictions are needed for accurate testing.

4. **Stool:** A stool microbiology test can be used to detect and identify various bacteria and yeasts that cause infection in the lower digestive tract. These tests can be done by the lab or a kit can be sent home for you to fill and then sent to the lab where they will do a microscopic examination. Yeast is normally found in very small amounts in the lower intestinal tract. A normal finding would contain almost none to very small amounts of yeast, however, if there is few,moderate to many found it is considered abnormal and signs of a Candida Overgrowth

5. **Blood:** A blood test will most likely only be done for diagnosis of systemic Candida that has entered the bloodstream. A blood test tests for antibodies produced by the body to combat bacteria, viruses and invaders like Candida. It is important to note that blood testing can provide false positives and fake negatives and it is important to interpret it with a healthcare professional.

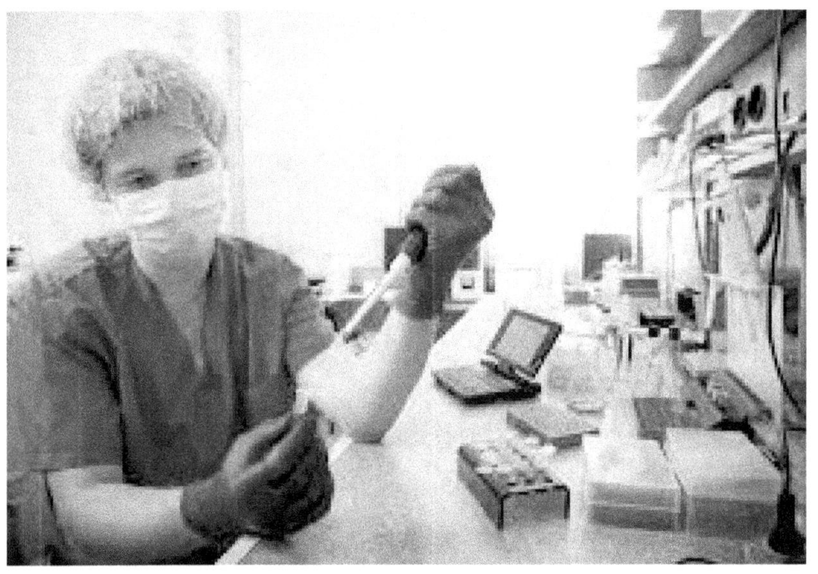

6

Candida and Other Health Conditions

Candida's implications can go further than its immediate effects and can exacerbate other health issues, specifically digestive disorders and skin conditions. It is important to understand the knock on effect of Candida overgrowth and how it often further affects other issues.

Candida overgrowth disrupts the gut balance and can exacerbate autoimmune disorders also. Acknowledging this underscores the importance of maintaining a healthy gut balance to manage Candida and help alleviate symptoms of underlying autoimmune disorders and improve overall immune function.

The Gut-Immune Connection:

Emerging research suggests a potential link between Candida overgrowth and autoimmune diseases. Disruption of the gut microbiome, often associated with Candida overgrowth, can trigger immune responses that may contribute to autoimmune conditions. Conditions such as inflammatory bowel disease (IBD), rheumatoid arthritis, and psoriasis have been studied for potential connections to Candida overgrowth.

Understanding the intricate interplay between Candida, the gut microbiome, and the immune system is an ongoing area of research that may provide insights into the development and management of autoimmune diseases.

It's important to collaborate with healthcare professionals for accurate diagnosis and tailored treatment plans when addressing Candida-related concerns or potential connections to other health conditions.

III

Treating Candida

7

Conventional Medical Approaches

I n the realm of conventional medicine a key avenue for the treatment of Candida is the use of antifungal medicines. These medicines are designed to target the Candida directly through a variety of mechanisms of action depending on the type and severity of the infection, the patient's overall health and drug responsiveness. Here is a concise overview of the most common types of antifungal medications.

1. **Oral Antifungals (fluconazole, itraconazole, and ketoconazole):** Oral antifungals are taken by mouth in the form of tablets or capsules. They are designed to be absorbed into the bloodstream, allowing them to circulate throughout the body to target fungal infections systemically. These medications are often prescribed for widespread or more severe Candida infections.

2. **Topical Antifungals (clotrimazole, miconazole, and nystatin):** Topical antifungal medications are applied directly to the affected area of the skin or mucous membranes. They are effective for localized fungal infections, such as oral thrush or skin-related Candida infections like athlete's foot. Common topical antifungals

include clotrimazole, miconazole, and nystatin.

3. **Intravenous (IV) Antifungals (amphotericin B and caspofungin):** In cases of severe or systemic Candida infections, IV antifungals are administered directly into the bloodstream through a vein. This method ensures that the medication reaches high concentrations in the body, effectively targeting the infection. IV antifungals like amphotericin B and caspofungin are often used in hospital settings for critically ill patients.

4. **Combination Therapies:** In many cases a combination of antifungal medications might be prescribed to enhance efficacy. This approach is especially useful for addressing complexes and resistant Candida infections.

When addressing Candida with conventional medicine it is always necessary to consult a healthcare professional in order to determine the best approach and to monitor for any side effects or complications.

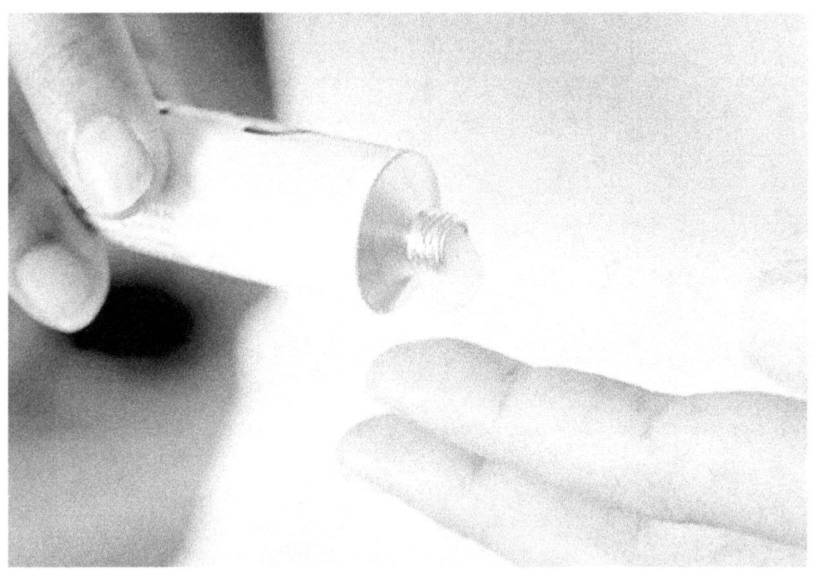

8

Holistic Healing Strategies

The Holistic approach is crucial to any treatment approach when it comes to Candida. Implementing herbal supplementation and making sure to include Candida Fighting foods into your diet, introducing pre- & probiotics is cornerstone to fighting Candida but also reducing stress and getting ample sleep. Below are some herbal remedies that help fight or reduce symptoms of Candidiasis.

<u>Natural Remedies for Candida</u>

Prebiotics & Probiotics: Where Probiotics are live bacteria that are found in certain food products that promote a healthy gut microbiome, Prebiotics are the food that these bacteria eat. So including a synbiotics combination of both is crucial to treating Candidiasis. It is recommended to discuss the use with a nutritionist as some approaches, depending on severity, type and the client, will at first not include any synbiotics until it is time to rebuild the gut microbiome. Some to consider are:

Saccharomyces boulardii

Lactobacillus acidophilus

Lactobacillus paracasei

Lactobacillus plantarum

- Bacillus subtilis
- Lactobacillus helvecticus
- Bifidobacterium

Hebs & Essential oil: There is a wide ranging list of plant allies to introduce to help fight everything from inflammation, fungal growth and immune function. These foods can be used as essential oils in localized applications or ingest as herbs, teas etc. Some herbs to introduce would be:

- Garlic,
- Tea tree oil
- Thyme
- Grapefruit seed extract
- Cinnamon
- Ginger
- Oregano
- Peppermint
- Berberine
- Caprylic Acid
- Rosemary

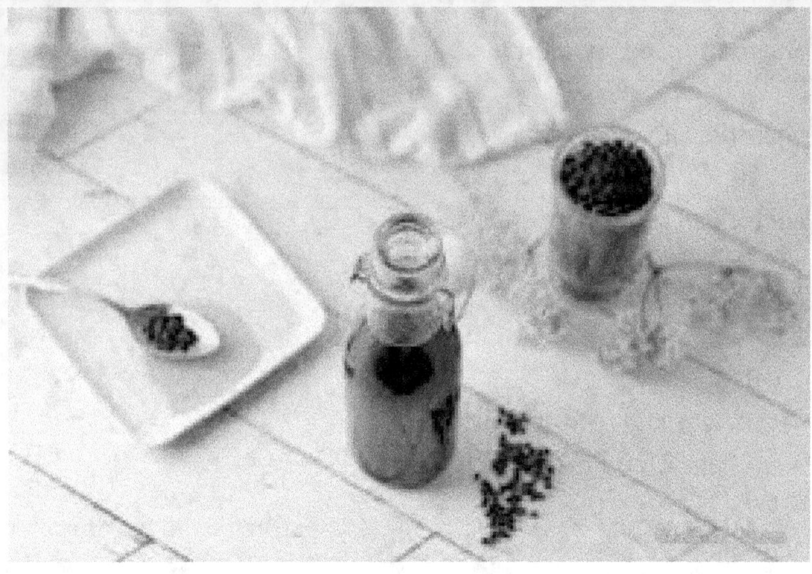

Teas: The leaves, bark & flowers and plants and trees all have a variety of functions against Candida. Teas to consider are:

- Chamomile
- Dandelion root
- Ginger
- Turmeric
- Peppermint
- Pau d'arco
- Burdock

Other foods, minerals, nutrients: There are many other foods and minerals that really help fight Candida in their own way. For example:

- Apple Cider vinegar is antifungal and helps with gut ph.
- Coconut Oil contains MCT's like Caprylic Acid which are antifungal, antimicrobial and antiviral.
- Hydrogen Peroxide is antiseptic and kills bacteria and yeast.
- Vitamins B, C, D, E help with Immune function, antifungal, inflammation and soothing the skin..

There is a broad spectrum of natural products available to help combat Candida and any good treatment protocol will elicit the help of Candida fighting Foods and Supplements.

IV

Lifestyle and Prevention

9

Lifestyle Changes

Candida overgrowth is a condition that is influenced as you now know by many factors including diet, lifestyle, and stress levels. Adopting a proactive approach to lifestyle and prevention is key in managing a healthy gut balance and a good healthy Candida balance. After treating a Candida overgrowth and managing to stabilize gut health and Candida levels it is then important to continue some practices and being conscious of your lifestyle and diet to not encourage overgrowth again. Establishing long term habits and diet is what is necessary to maintain health and vitality.

Maintaining Candida Balance takes and ongoing and conscious eye on our diet and consumption, with the purpose of maintaining a healthy Micro community.

Preventing Candida Overgrowth requires maintaining a healthy body & immune system, keeping inflammation low, and keeping up on sleep and low on Stress. Once the gut is balanced these factors are the underlying cause of overgrowth again so must also be managed as far as an ongoing lifestyle change is considered. Creating a healthy, pH balanced, allergen & toxin free, inflammation free, and food minimal prevents Candida from thriving and taking over again.

We have covered some dietary modifications but when it comes to management of Candida, Immune System, Inflammation this is where certain foods need to be fully integrated into daily routine and below is an example of some.

Foods to still include regularly are:

- Live Yogurt, Kefir
- Fermented foods like Kimchi, Sauerkraut.
- Apple cider vinegar
- Almonds
- Olive oil, Coconut oil
- Kombucha (beware for sugar in commercial products)
- Garlic, Ginger, Cloves

Candida being part of the natural microbiome it needs to be monitored and kept in balance. With so many factors influencing it these habits and dietary changes need to become lifestyle changes that are fully incorporated.

That Includes amongst others:

- Dietary Modifications
- Stress Reduction
- Inflammation Reduction
- Sleep Improvement

- Physical Workout Routine
- Detox Routine
- Hygiene Practices
- Hydration
- Alcohol consumption reduction

Fully integrating this into your life will not only help with Candida symptoms but will have overlapping benefits for your overall health and well-being.

V

Recap Overview: Action steps for Diet, Nutrition and Lifestyle Changes.

Action steps for Diet, Nutrition and Lifestyle Changes.

Managing Candida requires a comprehensive approach that takes into consideration diet, nutrition and lifestyle changes. Below we recap some action steps and an overview of the basic principles to keep in mind for fighting Candida overgrowth.

Dietary Modifications:

- Reduce sugars - Limit the intake of sugars, specifically refined sugars, sweet foods, desserts and only include low sugar fruit if any.
- Minimize Carbohydrates - Cut back on processed foods and refined grains and rather opt for whole grains like wild rice, quinoa and whole wheat
- Focus Whole foods - Prioritize nutrient rich vegetable, lean proteins and healthy fats
- Include antifungal food - Incorporate garlic, ginger, coconut oil and other anti-fungal foods to your diet.
- Avoid allergens - Avoid Dairy and gluten and other inflammatory

foods.
- Stay Hydrated – Drink plenty of water to support digestion and toxin elimination.

Nutritional Support:

- Prebiotics – Include prebiotic supplementation into your diet including Consume foods like ginger, garlic, asparagus, dandelion root, chicory all help with gut health and
- Probiotics – Include high quality probiotic supplements to encourage gut microbiome diversity and health.
- Fermented foods – Include fermented foods like live probiotic yogurt, kefir, sauerkraut, Kimchi into diet that naturally boost probiotic levels

Lifestyle Changes:

- Stress reduction – Reduce your stress levels and potentially include mindfulness practices and meditation to manage stress levels.
- Adequate sleep – Get adequate rest and sleep for improved immune function and emotional wellbeing
- Physical activity – Regular exercise enhances circulation, mood and overall health
- Hygiene practices – Maintain good hygiene, especially in areas prone to candida/fungal growth.

Other preventive measures:

- Avoid Alcohol to avoid its negative impact on gut health
- Antibiotic awareness, only use antibiotics when absolutely necessary and prescribed by a healthcare professional.
- Regular check-ups are useful to keep track of your overgrowth and progress.

As you take on these Action steps remember it is a process and you should listen to your body, be patient and make gradual changes that work for you. While these changes target Candida specifically they will also improve overall health, vitality and well being. Empower yourself with knowledge and a commitment to self care as you navigate this transformative journey

11

Conclusion

As we conclude this comprehensive look at Candida and its intricate role in human health, it is important to reflect on the profound impact that Candida overgrowth can have on our health and well-being. From digestive disruptions to skin discomfort and even potential risks of broader health conditions. Candida's influence is far reaching but with knowledge and understanding, and the tools to take action, we can take control back.

We've delved into the nuances of Candida biology, its interactions within the body, and the array of symptoms it can evoke. We've explored the dynamic relationship between diet, gut health, and Candida balance, realizing the power of our choices.

With proactive steps such as embracing a balanced diet, incorporating probiotics, managing stress and being

If you have enjoyed reading this book and found it to be helpful on your journey fighting and managing Candida I'd be very appreciative if you could leave a favorable review for the book on Amazon.

VI

Conclusion, Appendices, Resources

12

Conclusion

As we conclude this comprehensive look at Candida and its intricate role in human health, it is important to reflect on the profound impact that Candida overgrowth can have on our health and well-being. From digestive disruptions to skin discomfort and even potential risks of broader health conditions. Candida's influence is far reaching but with knowledge and understanding, and the tools to take action, we can take control back.

We've delved into the nuances of Candida biology, its interactions within the body, and the array of symptoms it can evoke. We've explored the dynamic relationship between diet, gut health, and Candida balance, realizing the power of our choices.

With proactive steps such as embracing a balanced diet, incorporating probiotics, managing stress and being

If you have enjoyed reading this book and found it to be helpful on your journey fighting and managing Candida I'd be very appreciative if you could leave a favorable review for the book on Amazon.

13

Appendices

<u>Anti-Candida Food Plan Guidelines</u>

In general foods are restricted because of their Carbohydrate (sugar) content. Legumes might be a good source of protein but due to being very starchy they are also avoided. Peanuts and pistachios are to be avoided due to their high mold content, which can exacerbate Candida. Mushrooms are a fungus and may also cross react with Candida. Fermented foods like vinegars and aged cheese may also provoke symptoms because of the similarities to candida and may feeds candida yeasts. Fermented foods like kefir, and sauerkraut may also be beneficial to gut health however it is recommended to eliminate them at first and gradually introduce them into your diet. The following modifications are to be implemented at least 2-4 weeks to reset gut health and the slowly introducing and maintaining healthy gut foods, but as the approach may change from person to person it is recommended to assess with your healthcare professional which foods to include/exclude out of your specific diet. These modifications are usually followed for a 2-4 week period to assess personal response.

Category	To Include	To Exclude
Fruit	Low sugar fruit like Cherries, Dark Berries, Lemons, Limes, Avocado, Coconut & Grapefruit	Bananas, Pineapple, Papaya, all dried fruits and juices
Egg, Dairy, & diary replacement	Eggs, Unsweetened live probiotic yogurt, hemp milk, unsweetened coconut milk.	Milk & Milk substitutes, all aged cheeses.
Grains	100% Whole grains only like Wild Rice, Quinoa, Barley, Rye, Buckwheat, Whole Spelt, etc. 1 serving per day maximum.	All refined grains, breads, sweetened baked goods
Animal Protein	Fish (Fresh or Canned) & other seafood, Chicken, Turkey, Lean Beef, Pork, Lamb (preferably pasture raised on natural organic diets) 1-2 Servings per day	Processed meats & Cold Cuts
Fats & Oils	Avocado, Ghee, Cold Pressed Oil of: Olive, Coconut, Avocado, sesame, pumpkin seed.	Margarine, Shortening, Processed oils, prepared salad dressings, spreads, sauces, and mayonnaise
Vegetables	Non-Starchy vegetables - raw, steamed, sauteed, grilled, baked and juiced	Mushrooms, Potatoes, Sweet potatoes and Corn
Nuts & Seeds	Walnuts, Hazelnuts, Pecans, Almonds, Cashews, Macadamia, Flax Seed, Pumpkin seed, Sunflower seed, Poppy seeds, Sesame seed - whole nut butters	Peanuts & Pistachios including peanut & pistachio nut butters
Acidic & Fermented Foods	Lemon & Lime	All Vinegars and preserved foods, Sauerkraut, Pickles, and other foods preserved in brine or vinegar
Sweeteners	Stevia as a herbal sweetener	All white/brown sugars, honey, maple, agave, corn syrup of any kind, molasses, brown rice syrup, fruit sweeteners
Beverages	Filtered, Spring or Distilled water (lots), herbal teas (chamomile, bergamot, lemon grass, ginger, pau d' arco, dandelion	Sodas, Alcohol, coffee & caffeine, creamers.

Depending on the approach taken by you and your health practitioner a simpler but stricter approach would be to remove:

- **All Grains**
- **All Fruit**
- **All Dairy, except for Live Probiotic Whole Yogurt**

This would be done at very least for 2-4 weeks and if no clear results in symptoms is felt yet you're to continue another 7-14 days at a time until the symptoms disappear and have not returned either.

Once your initial reset is done careful consideration needs to be taken with the reintroduction of foods. The gut balance can easily be disrupted and so it is important to slowly add foods one by one to assess sensitivity and response and also to build a strong gut biome. Here is a simple food reintroduction guideline to follow.

Food Re-introductions

At the end of the additional 7-14 days, please add the above 3 food groups into your diet, very gradually,

Day 1: add 1 serving (1/2 cup) whole grain daily, such as quinoa, brown or wild rice. After 3-4 days on grains, assess symptoms and if well tolerated with little or no digestive symptoms (or other symptoms that had been bothering you), add the next food group below. If not well tolerated, stay on just the grains for several more days until tolerance improves. It is best to do this as slowly as needed.

Day 3 or 4: add 1 fruit, such as orange or apple, each day. After 3-4 more days, assess symptoms. If well tolerated, proceed to the next food. If not well-tolerated repeat the above procedure by waiting several more days.

Day 7 or 8: add a dairy product, such as cottage cheese, or ricotta. Continue to assess symptoms and report to your healthcare practitioner. You may

Meal Plan Recipe Suggestions

The following are menu suggestions. Since this meal plan is quite low in carbohydrates, you may experience cravings at first, but this will pass and you will soon feel quite satisfied. If you are hungry you may increase your portion size since this is not a calorie-restricted program. Any recipe may be used for any meal; leftovers from dinner make a quick lunch. However on a Candida control diet it is best to use leftovers within 24 hours or discard.

Breakfast Ideas

1. Scrambled Eggs with Spinach and Garlic
2. Chia Seed Pudding with Stevia and Berries
3. Greek Yogurt with Fresh Berries
4. Vegetable Omelet with Herbs and Spices
5. Smoothie Bowl with Spinach, Avocado, and Berries
6. Avocado and Smoked Salmon on Whole Grain Rice Cakes
7. Coconut Flour Pancakes with Stevia
8. Almond Butter and Celery Sticks
9. Millet Porridge with Cinnamon and Almonds
10. Herbal Tea with Lemon and a Boiled Egg
11. Sardines on Whole Grain Crackers with Cucumber and Tomato Slices

Lunch Ideas

1. Grilled Chicken Salad with Mixed Greens and Veggies
2. Quinoa and Vegetable Stir-Fry with Low-Sugar Sauce
3. Tuna Salad Lettuce Wraps
4. Cauliflower Rice Bowl with Veggies and Protein

5. Zucchini Noodles with Pesto
6. Avocado and Turkey Lettuce Wraps
7. Egg Salad on Cucumber Slices
8. Creamy Mushroom and Spinach Soup
9. Baked Salmon with Roasted Vegetables
10. Cabbage and Ground Turkey Stir-Fry
11. Broccoli and Almond Soup
12. Tofu and Vegetable Skewers with Low-Sugar Marina

Dinner Ideas

1. Grilled Salmon with Lemon and Dill, Steamed Broccoli, and Quinoa or Cauliflower Rice
2. Stir-Fried Tofu and Vegetables with Coconut Aminos or Tamari, Served with Cauliflower Rice
3. Baked Chicken Thighs with Herbs, Sautéed Spinach, and Roasted Brussels Sprouts
4. Cauliflower Crust Pizza with Sugar-Free Tomato Sauce, Veggies, and Optional Cheese
5. Grilled Shrimp Skewers with Olive Oil and Garlic Marinade, Alongside Bell Peppers and Zucchini
6. Zoodle (Zucchini Noodle) Primavera with Cherry Tomatoes, Garlic, Basil, and Optional Chicken or Tofu
7. Lemon Herb Baked Cod with Asparagus and a Mixed Greens Salad
8. Cabbage and Ground Beef Casserole with Tomato Sauce
9. Mushroom and Spinach Stuffed Chicken Breast, Served with Roasted Cauliflower and a Light Cream Sauce
10. Spaghetti Squash with Pesto and Grilled Chicken
11. Baked Eggplant Parmesan with Almond Flour Coating, Tomato Sauce, and Sautéed Greens
12. Thai-Inspired Coconut Curry with Tofu, Bell Peppers, and Broccoli,

Served Over Cauliflower Rice

55

14

Resources

- Beeson, K. (2023). Which Probiotics are Best for Candida? *Professionals.* https://www.optibacprobiotics.com/professionals/latest-re search/gut-health/probiotics-best-for-candida
- C De Oliveira Santos, G., C Vasconcelos, C., J.O. Lopes, A., S. De Sousa Cartagenes, M. D., K.D.B. Filho, A., R.F. Do Nascimento, F., M. Ramos, R., R.R.B. Pires, E., S. De Andrade, M., M.G. Rocha, F., & De Andrade Monteiro, C. (2018). Candida Infections and Therapeutic Strategies: Mechanisms of Action for Traditional and Alternative Agents. *PubMed Central*, PMC6038711.
- Charlie. (2022, March 6). 5 ways to test for candida | Kolorex® blog. *Natural Herbs for Candida - Kolorex Natural Anti-candida Support.* https://www.kolorex.com/knowledge/five-ways-to-test-for-cand ida
- Cohen, M. (2023). Candida Test: Everything You Need To Know About Candidiasis Testing. *The IBS & Gut Health Clinic.* https://ibsgu thealthclinic.co.uk/candida-test/
- Hidalgo, J. A., MD. (n.d.). *Candidiasis treatment & management: medical care, surgical care, consultations.* https://emedicine.meds

cape.com/article/213853-treatment?form=fpf

- Kunde, R. (2021, December 14). *What to know about candidiasis tests.* WebMD. https://www.webmd.com/skin-problems-and-treatments/what-to-know-candidiasis-tests
- Ld, A. E. M. R. (2023, March 16). *The Candida Diet: Beginner's Guide and Meal Plan.* Healthline. https://www.healthline.com/nutrition/candida-diet
- Migala, J. (2022, February 8). *Candida Diet 101: Beginner's Guide, Detailed food List, 7-Day Meal Plan.* EverydayHealth.com. https://www.everydayhealth.com/diet-nutrition/candida-diet-beginners-guide-detailed-food-list-meal-plan/
- Ohshima, T., Kojima, Y., J Seneviratne, C., & Maeda, N. (2016). Therapeutic Application of Synbiotics, a Fusion of Probiotics and Prebiotics, and Biogenics as a New Concept for Oral Candida Infections: A Mini Review. *PubMed Central.* https://www.ncbi.nlm.nih.gov/pmc/articles/PMC4724717/
- Rd, S. L. (2023, February 14). *Probiotics and prebiotics: what's the difference?* Healthline. https://www.healthline.com/nutrition/probiotics-and-prebiotics

About the Author

Cornelius Muller has been a reader on all things health, nutrition, lifestyle and well-being but having been struggling with Candidiasis for years and finally sitting down to study the issue he found that the topics is shrouded in mystery and direction. This lead Cornelius to write a book that is comprehensive yet concise and short format for anybody interested in the topic of Candida or struggling with Candida to be able to equip themselves with the basic understanding of Candida, its functions, defenses and how to attack and treat it. This book is the culmination of those events.